Handbook of

MEDICAL SOCIOLOGY

for Nursing, Physiotherapy and Paramedical Students

Handbook of MEDICAL SOCIOLOGY for Nursing, Physiotherapy and Paramedical Students

Varun Malhotra MBBS MD (Community Medicine)
Department of Community Medicine
Kamineni Institute of Medical Sciences
Narketpally, Nalgonda, Andhra Pradesh, India

Ritika Malhotra
MA (Economics) PG Dip (Health and Family Welfare)
Health Educator
Malhotra Nursing Home
Panchkula, Haryana, India

JAYPEE BROTHERS MEDICAL PUBLISHERS (P) LTD

New Delhi • London • Philadelphia • Panama

Jaypee Brothers Medical Publishers (P) Ltd.

Headquarters

Jaypee Brothers Medical Publishers (P) Ltd.
4838/24, Ansari Road, Daryaganj
New Delhi 110 002, India
Phone: +91-11-43574357
Fax: +91-11-43574314
Email: jaypee@jaypeebrothers.com

Overseas Offices

J.P. Medical Ltd.
83, Victoria Street, London
SW1H 0HW (UK)
Phone: +44-2031708910
Fax: +02-03-0086180
Email: info@jpmedpub.com

Jaypee-Highlights Medical Publishers Inc.
City of Knowledge, Bld. 237, Clayton
Panama City, Panama
Phone: +507-301-0496
Fax: +507-301-0499
Email: cservice@jphmedical.com

Jaypee Brothers Medical Publishers Ltd.
The Bourse
111, South Independence Mall East
Suite 835, Philadelphia
PA 19106, USA
Phone: + 267-519-9789
Email: joe.rusko@jaypeebrothers.com

Jaypee Brothers Medical Publishers (P) Ltd.
17/1-B Babar Road, Block-B
Shaymali, Mohammadpur
Dhaka-1207, Bangladesh
Mobile: +08801912003485
Email: jaypeedhaka@gmail.com

Jaypee Brothers Medical Publishers (P) Ltd.
Shorakhute
Kathmandu, Nepal
Phone: +00977-9841528578
Email: jaypee.nepal@gmail.com

Website: www.jaypeebrothers.com
Website: www.jaypeedigital.com

Inquiries for bulk sales may be solicited at: jaypee@jaypeebrothers.com

Handbook of Medical Sociology for Nursing, Physiotherapy and Paramedical Students

First Edition: **2013**, Reprint: **2023**

ISBN 978-93-5090-513-5

Printed in India

Dedicated to

Dr (Brig) MK Ghosh (Retd)
Professor and Head
Department of Community Medicine
and
Students of
Bachelor of Physiotherapy
Sikkim Manipal Institute of Medical Sciences
Tadong, Sikkim, India

Preface

There is no dearth of books on Sociology. However, there is need for many more because the subject is wide and varied. Every family is unique, every village has its own culture and every state has its own language. This book does not attempt to fulfill that requirement. As name (and size) of the book aptly indicates, it is not a treatise on the subject. The objective of the book is neither to wean medical and paramedical students away from in-depth study of the subject nor to prevent learning it through interactive sessions in the classrooms. No book can take away the role of a teacher. Still every examination system requires a handbook that a student needs to revise the subject. The book aims to fill that gap. We would like to make the book more user-friendly, and for that suggestions and criticism from the readers are more than welcome.

Varun Malhotra
Ritika Malhotra

Acknowledgments

We express, sincere gratitude to our parents and teachers. We also learnt from our families, friends, colleagues and many by whom, we had opportunity to work, play and walk with. We are grateful to all 'these and those'. The real learning is in classroom, and we understand, one learns better when he/she is on the other side of podium; hence our indebtness to our students.

No author forgets his first publisher; we also will not. Our acknowledgment to Shri Jitendar P Vij (Group Chairman), Mr Ankit Vij (Managing Director), Mr Tarun Duneja (Director-Publishing), Mrs Samina Khan (PA to Director-Publishing), Mr KK Raman (Production Manager), Mr Sunil Kumar Dogra (Production Executive), Mr Neelambar Pant (Production Coordinator), Dr Mohd Naved (Senior Proofreader), Rakesh Kumar (Typesetter) and other staff of M/s Jaypee Brothers Medical Publishers (P) Ltd, New Delhi, India, for their untiring efforts.

Contents

Sociology and Its Relevance to Medical Sciences

chapter 1

Definition

Sociology is the scientific study of societies: Study of human behavior, and relationships between human beings. Medical sociology deals mainly with social factors that are related with health and disease.

Relevance of medical sociology

Study of sociology is relevant and important for future doctors, nurses, physiotherapists and other paramedics, both for diagnosis and management of patients. It is, as important to know *who we are treating*, as *what we are treating*. Relevance of Sociology for students of medical, nursing and physiotherapy are as follows:

- **World Health Organization** has defined health as "a state of complete physical, **social** and mental well being, and not merely an absence of disease or infirmity". As per this definition social well being of an individual is as important as physical or mental well being.
- It is now well appreciated that health of individuals and community, and occurrences of diseases are intimately related with social factors, e.g. type of **family, community** (rural or urban), **culture**, religion, folk-ways, mores, life style, etc. These aspects are learnt through process of **socialization**, in primary and secondary **social groups**.
- **Social control** operating through informal or formal means has significant influence on health behavior of members

of community. Recent technological innovations like TV, internet, affordable two-wheelers, etc. have brought about significant **social changes** that have implications on health of individuals and community.

- Changing **status and roles** of women in Indian society in recent decades has affected all aspects of human life, including health.
- One of the pillars of primary health care is community participation. Community participation can be best achieved if we are aware of community; its leaders, customs, taboos, etc. In short, if we want the community to participate in our march towards Health for All, we have to know **community**.
- Determinants of health, e.g. nutrition, environmental health etc. are all related with culture, and human behavior.
- **Life style** is gaining important role in causation of modern diseases, e.g. obesity, IHD, Diabetes, cancers and HIV/AIDS.
- **Social leaders** have been recognized as valuable resources for brining about positive changes in health behavior of individuals and groups.
- **Social pathology** deals with social factors responsible for diseases. Poverty, illiteracy, and ignorance are factors that are closely related with incidence and prevalence of diseases.
- Studies have shown that there are difference in incidence and prevalence of diseases, mortality rates and pattern of diseases in different **Social Classes**.
- It has now been well recognized that availability of health services is not the only answer to prevention. Health services should be acceptable and affordable by the people who need them the most.
- **Social Security** is closely related to provision of comprehensive health services.

- Health related legislations need an understanding of **society** as well as medical aspects of the disease.
- **Medicosocial problems** like delinquency, prostitution, crimes, beggary, etc. have medical implications. These require combined and coordinated involvement of medical and social agencies as well as State.
- Similarly many medical problems like care of handicapped, old people, etc. can not be addressed, unless there is active involvement of society.
- **NGOs** have in many fields of public health have achieved what the Government machinery could not. Example family planning, HIV/AIDS, care of disabled. The lesson learnt is that better understanding of community is essential for achieving our health related aims and objectives.
- Health Indicators of Kerala are better than many richer states of our Nation. It is believed that high literacy rate especially of women is an important determinant of health.
- Diet is an integral part of culture and its modification is an important aspect in many diseases example obesity, diabetes, malnutrition, etc.

Society

chapter

2

Definition

In general usage 'society' means group of people. However, in Sociology, the term 'society' refers, not to group of people, **but relationships between them**. It is the system of relationship that exists between individuals of the group. Society is also defined as a web of social relationships.

Characteristics of society

a. Social Order. Social order is maintained through formal and informal social control.
b. Likeness is essential prerequisite of Society.
c. Interdependence.
d. Co-operation.

Types of society

Tribal society

Tribe is a group of persons having:

i. Common territory
ii. Common language
iii. Blood relationship (Kinship)
iv. Endogamy, i.e. marriages within the tribe
v. Political Organization
vi. Importance of religion
vii. Common name.

Important features of tribal society

i. Main economic activity is hunting and food gathering.
ii. Division of labor is minimal, and is based on gender and age. There is no specialization.
iii. No private property, i.e. property is common to all members of tribe.
iv. Primary group
v. Folkways and mores are important means of social control.
vi. Small and homogeneous in composition.

Agrarian society

i. Dominant economic activity is agriculture.
ii. Characteristics of rural community.
iii. Minimal division of labor.
iv. Family plays an important role.
v. Sense of unity, 'we feeling'.
vi. Social control is through informal means.
vii. Simplicity, homogeneity and close-ness to nature.

Industrial society

i. Emergence of modern family.
ii. Manufacture and service are dominant economic activities.
iii. Division of labor (specialization) is pronounced.
iv. Multiple roles
v. Impersonal relationships.
vi. Class vs caste. Class is more important than caste.
vii. Social mobility is feasible.
viii. **Status of women:** Women are economically and socially more independent.

Community

chapter

3

Definition

Community is a group of people living in a limited geographical area, having common and inter-dependent life.

Main characteristics of community

i. Community is a group of people, sharing basic conditions of common life.
ii. **Locality:** Community has definite locality.
iii. **Community sentiments:** Feeling of belonging together.
iv. Permanency.
v. **Naturality:** Communities are not act of will, but natural. One is born into a community.
vi. **Likeness:** In community, there is likeness in language, customs, mores etc.
vii. **Wider Ends:** Members of a community associate for wider ends (not a particular end).
viii. **Identity:** Community has a name, an identity.
ix. Community has no legal status.
x. Important differences between society and community are tabulated in Table 3.1.

Rural community

i. **Cultural homogeneity:** Activities, needs, aspirations, behavior, etc. of most natives of villages are similar.

Table 3.1: Differences between Society and Community

Society	*Community*
There is an element of likeness in society, but it is not necessary the feeling of oneness	To constitute a community, the presence of community sentiment (we feeling) among its members is must
Society has no defined boundary	Community has defined geographical boundary
Society is a larger group	There are many communities in a society
Society is abstract concept	Community is concrete concept
Society as a group is 'means to an end'	Community as a group is 'end in itself'

ii. **Self dependence and reliance:** The members of rural community are able to fulfill most of their demands by themselves.
iii. Rural community is smaller, and members know each other by face, name, caste etc.
iv. **Caste system is very strong in rural community:** Social status is dependent on caste.
v. **Cooperation and conflict:** Both cooperation and conflict are present. On one hand all festivals/ceremonies are attended by whole village, however, conflicts on land/water/caste, etc. are not uncommon.
vi. **Social unity:** There is 'WE' feeling among rural community. Outside his village, an individual is recognized by his village.
vii. **Lack of social mobility:** Lack of social mobility is an important feature of rural life.
viii. Status of females is still low. Female literacy in rural India is dismally low. Pardah custom is still prevalent in rural India.

ix. **Conservative society:** Not willing for social change.
x. Joint families.
xi. Religion plays an important part in life of rural community.

Urban community

i. Artificial ways of life.
ii. Industries and Services are main occupations.
iii. Cultural heterogeneity.
iv. Urban areas are dependent upon other cities and rural areas for their needs.
v. Urban areas are larger in size, have more number of people, and higher population density.
vi. Caste system is weak. Class system is more importance.
vii. Cooperation is almost absent in cities. Services have to be purchased.
viii. 'I' feeling. Individuals are recognized by his class, status, role etc.
ix. Social mobility is a way of life.
x. Females in urban areas have more freedom to acquire education and take up jobs.
xi. Modern and progressive society. Social changes are feasible.
xii. Nuclear families.
xiii. Religion plays lesser role in community life of urban India.

Important differences between rural and urban communities are tabulated in Table 3.2.

Impact of industrialization and urbanization on health

Urban population has increased from 10.84 percent in 1901 to 27.8 percent in 2001. Reasons for urbanization are:

a. Industrialization provides direct and indirect employment to thousands. This draws rural people to urban areas.

Table 3.2: Differences between rural and urban community		
Characteristics	*Rural*	*Urban*
Relationship	Personal, we feeling	Impersonal, I feeling
Family	Joint	Nuclear
Marriage	Arranged, divorce rare	Love marriages not uncommon; increasing divorce rates
Status of women	Lower	Higher, more economic independence
Social control	Through informal means	Formal control
Division of labor	Less	More pronounced
Caste & class system	Caste system	Class system
Role of religion	More	Less
Way of life	Homogeneous	Heterogeneous
Social mobility	Less (caste system)	More (class system)
Occupation	Agricultural	Industry, service (office jobs)
Status	By birth (caste system)	Acquired
Moral values	Higher	Lower, moral laxity
Type of life	Less dynamic	Dynamic, fast
Personality	Balanced	Higher rates of personality disorders
Crime rates	Less	Higher
Size	Small	Large
Density	Low	High density
Facilities	Lower	Higher facilities for education, transport, entertainment, etc.

b. Better facilities for education, communication, entertainment, i.e. better quality of life.
c. Natural disasters displace people to urban areas.
d. Social discrimination on basis of caste, gender etc. is less is urban areas.

Disadvantages of unplanned urbanization

However influx of rural people to cities has many disadvantages. Unplanned urbanization means more slums, where quality of life is poor, social control is lacking and legal machinery may be ineffective. These factors lead to deterioration of physical, social and mental health of people who have migrated from rural areas to slums.

Environmental degradation

i. Unsafe water supply
ii. Unsanitary disposal of human and animal wastes
iii. Overcrowding
iv. Breeding of vectors
v. Industrial waste causing air and water pollution
vi. Noise pollution due to industry, air traffic.
vii. Industrial accidents e.g. Bhopal Gas Tragedy, radiation accidents
viii. Smoke nuisance in homes.

Communicable diseases

i. Higher rates of water and food borne disease.
ii. Higher morbidity due to infections related with overcrowding e.g. tuberculosis.
iii. Higher incidence of vector borne diseases e.g. malaria, dengue
iv. Higher incidence of sexually transmitted diseases.

Noncommunicable diseases

Unhealthy life styles in slums i.e. lack of exercise, more dependence on high calorie foods, smoking, consumption of alcohol and mental stress raise the risk of hypertension, diabetes and coronary artery disease.

Food sanitation: Poor environmental conditions, lack of facilities for personal hygiene and dependence on out of home kitchens for meals mean poor food sanitation and higher rates of diseases transmitted through food.

Accidents: Accidents rates due to road traffic accidents and home accidents are higher in slums.

Mental health: Higher rates of accidents, homicides, crimes, drug and alcohol addictions are evidences that mental health deteriorates in slums.

Social health: Lack of family life and social control are important reasons for declining social health in slums. Increase in crime rates, prostitution, extra-marital relations, child abuse, drug and alcohol consumption, gender violence, etc. are examples.

Increase morbidity and mortality: Due to above reasons and accidents.

Advantages of urbanization on health

i. Better medical facilities are available in urban areas.
ii. Better Communication e.g. telephone, road communication means faster availability of health Services.
iii. Better Educational facilities through formal and informal mean more awareness about prevention of diseases and advantages of seeking early treatment from qualified personnel.
iv. **Social security:** Employment in Government and industries means availability of medical services through

Social Security schemes e.g. CGHS, ESI, etc. for individuals as well as their families.

Conclusion

In brief, urbanization and industrialization are not bad for health of people. What is lacking is *planned urbanization*. Unregulated growth of cities leads to more slums where risks to health are more than in rural areas. To focus attention of the World on the issue, World Health Organization (WHO) declared its theme for World Health Day 2010 on April 7, 2010 as Urbanization—A challenge to Public Health.

Culture

chapter

4

Definition

Sir Edward Taylor has defined culture as 'that complex whole, which include knowledge, beliefs, norms, laws, religion, customs, skills and other capabilities acquired by an individual as a member of the society'.

Culture is also defined as a system of learned behavior shared by, and transmitted among the members of a group.

Important features of culture

- **Acquired:** Culture includes every thing learned by human beings in their life time, which is not inherited.
- **Shared:** Culture is shared by members of groups or society. It is not special to single individual.
- **Trans-generational:** Passed from one generation to next.

Structure of culture

i. Smallest part of culture is called 'culture trait'. Shaking hand or a wooden bowl is example of a trait.

ii. Traits combine to form cultural complexes. For example, Football complex include football, ground, players, rules, referee, audience, TV cameras, commentators, etc.

iii. Cultural complexes combine to form cultural pattern. For example industrial society is a cultural pattern. It has a way of life that is different from agricultural based society.

Components of culture

The principle components of culture are:

i. **Values:** Values are ideas and beliefs about what is "right" and what is "wrong". Values are not Do's and Don'ts, but guidelines for social behavior. Our value system gives more importance to religion, concern for others, etc. while in West success, achievements, etc. are more important. Thus values differ from society to society, as every social order chooses what is to be valued, and what is not.

ii. **Norms:** Norms are social rules which dictate correct and appropriate behavior in society. Norms tell what we must/should do, and what we must/should not do. Thus Norms are more explicit than values, and like Do's and Don'ts. Norms are enforced by sanctions, i.e. rewards and punishments. Norms can be further classified into Mores and Folkways (Table 4.1).

iii. **Folkways:**
   1. Customary ways of behavior
   2. Habits* those are common to group.
   3. Related with day to day way of behavior
   4. Socially approved
   5. Vary from society to society
   6. Followed automatically, spontaneously
   7. Not connected with moral values (unlike mores)
   8. If violated by an individual, he is ridiculed, laughed upon, boycotted (especially if violations are repeated)
   9. Examples: Way of greetings, way of dressing for an occasion, way of eating, standing, sitting, etc. Note that these examples satisfy all conditions mentioned above.

   **Note*-Habits are purely personal issues, not entailing obligation. For example having a bed tea, smoking, going for a walk in morning.

Table 4.1: Difference between Folkways and Mores	
Folkways	*Mores*
Customary way of behavior	Socially accepted behavior that involve moral values
Should be followed	Must be followed
Useful for day to day living	Essential for social welfare
Folkways change more rapidly	More deep rooted and change less rapidly
Followed spontaneously	Mores are more vigorously enforced
Followed not out of fear	Followed or avoided (Taboo) out of fear
Sanctions on violation of folkways are lenient	Sanctions on violation of mores are more strong
Vary from society to society, e.g. way of greeting differs among Hindus and Muslims	Being related with moral values, mores show less variation between societies Stealing is prohibited by all communities
For example ways of greeting, eating, dressing	Stealing, eve teasing, monogamy, incest, rape
Less likely to be converted into law	Mores often form basis for laws, e.g. Dowry Act

iv. **Mores:**
   1. Associated with moral values
   2. Society considers compliance with mores more important for its welfare, and maintenance of order.
   3. The reaction to violation is stronger (as compared to folk-ways)
   4. Negative mores (not to be done) are called taboos.
   5. More closely associated with law. Stealing is a taboo as well as crime. For example, stealing, eve teasing,

incest, misbehaviors with ladies, not returning loans, etc.

v. **Symbols and language:** Symbols are acts (e.g. gestures) or objects (e.g. flag) that have come to be socially accepted as standing for some particular thing. Language is the most important form of symbol. Language is a system of communication that uses sounds for structured meaning. Language is the chief vehicle by which people communicate ideas, information, attitudes and emotions. Language is the vehicle through which the culture is transmitted horizontally as well as vertically.

Role or functions of culture

Behavior of animals is based mainly on instincts. Babies of animals require little "learning" to become adults. But this is not the case with humans. A human baby is totally dependent on others, not only for its survival, but also for learning social behavior. We keep on learning during our infancy, childhood and adult life. What we learn is essential for our life in society because:

a. Culture makes a *Human* being out of a biological organism.
b. Culture provides us guidelines for day to day living.
c. Culture provides us a configuration of Do's and Don'ts.
d. Culture ensures stable social order.

Important terms

Cultural variability

Culture is not uniform, but varies from region to region. This is called cultural variability.

Cultural universality

Some aspects of culture are universal, e.g. family as a basic unit of society is present in all cultures.

Subculture

In each culture, we have subcultures, e.g. youth culture, working group culture.

Counter-culture

It is subculture that tries to oppose or reject many aspects of dominant culture. *Hippy movement* was an example of counter-culture.

Acculturation

Acculturation means cultural contact. When there is contact between people or group of people of different culture, there occurs diffusion of culture both ways. This is called acculturation.

Cultural Contact is promoted by:

i. Transportation and communication
ii. Trade and commerce. Globalization is promoting acculturation.
iii. Tourism
iv. Education
v. Media both electronic (TV and Internet) and print
vi. Propagation of religion.

Factors against cultural diffusion

Every society is a cultural island and it wants to safe guard against cultural invasion.

Physical isolation example tribal, sense of cultural superiority, taboos and cultural inertia also restrict acculturation.

Example of acculturation: Our dress or food habits have been influenced by Western world. Jeans, burgers, pizza, our language (slang, etc.) are leant through acculturation.

Advantages of acculturation: We have learnt science and technology from West. This has helped us to improve our quality of life.

Disadvantages of acculturation: For example, spread of tobacco use, fast foods are less healthy than home food.

Cultural Lag: Material aspects of culture (technological e.g. Internet) develop much rapidly than nonmaterial aspects (e.g. customs). This gap is called cultural lag and may be a cause for cultural conflicts or generation gap.

Culture in health and disease

Culture is closely related with health and disease. Many cultural factors are good for health; some are bad while most have no affect. Examples of some of the cultural practices that are related with health are given below:

Concept of etiology of disease

(a) Wrath of Gods (b) Sins of last birth (c) Evil or bad eye (d) Ghost entry (e) Bad food or water (f) Effect of climate, exposure to cold or heat (g)Impurity in blood.

Nutrition

Hot foods, e.g. nonvegetarian foods are considered hot food. Cold foods, e.g. curd, lemon juice etc. Hot foods are prohibited during fevers with rashes e.g. chicken pox. Cold foods are to be avoided in common cold. Milk is considered bad during productive cough.

Environmental sanitation

(a) Open defecation (b) Disposal of waste around houses (c) Water supply from pond where animals drink and bathe, and clothes, etc. are washed (d) *Katcha* houses, poor ventilation for security reason, absence of separate kitchen.

Personal hygiene

(a) Use of soil for hand washing (b) Regular bathing (c) Barber shaving using un-sterilized instruments (d) Purdah system increases incidence of TB (e) Not wearing footwear leads to hookworm infection (f) Sleeping on ground or outside increases in the incidence of insect/snake bites.

Food habits

(a) Vegetarian vs nonvegetarian (b) Some people do not eat onion/ garlic on religious grounds (c) All festivals and ceremonies have meals associated with them.

Mother and child health

(a) Women stays at home for 40 days after delivery (b) Special diet for pregnant women (c) Colostrum harmful for new borne (d) Prolonged breastfeeding practiced in India (e) Black spot (Tikka) to ward off evil eye.

Demography

(a) Universality of marriage (b) Early marriage (c) Dowry system (d) Male child preference.

Occupational health

Children following father occupation.

Organ-systems

Skin

Massage of skin with oil followed by exposure to the Sun—Vitamin D and good circulation of blood.

Eye

Sharing of needle to put *kajal* transmits infection like trachoma.

ENT

(a) Cleaning of ear by quacks leading to rupture of eardrum.
(b) Indiscriminate spitting causes spread of infection.

Oral health

(a) Regular brushing with Neem twig (b) Forceful mouthwash after meals is good habit (c) Tobacco chewing causes oral cancers.

Respiratory system

Smoking is bad habit. Use of *gobar* cakes as fuel in ill-ventilated houses leads to chronic bronchitis and COPD.

Social Groups

chapter

5

Social group is a collection of individuals in which there is:

a. Interaction among members on a regular basis.
b. The individual is conscious of belonging to the group.
c. Members share norms and values
d. There is interdependence, i.e. what happens to the group affects its members, and what happens to an individual affects other members.

Aggregates are collection of individuals who are in temporary physical proximity, but not in interaction. Two hundred people waiting at a railway station is an example of aggregate.

Statistical group is a group of people who have a common statistical feature, e.g. all individuals borne on September 7, 1978. In contrast **Social Category** is a group of people having a common acquired characteristic, e.g. all individuals speaking a particular language. In both, statistical group and social category, people are (a) not in proximity (b) there is no interaction among individuals.

Essential characteristics of social groups

1. Collection, i.e. two or more individuals
2. Interaction between members. This interaction may be direct or indirect.
3. Common interest or values or norms.
4. Being aware of belonging to the group
5. **Reciprocity:** It may be emotional or in action.

Classification of social groups

Primary and secondary groups: These will be discussed in detail later. Important differences between primary and secondary groups are tabulated in Table 5.1.

Permanent and temporary groups: For example, family (permanent) and crowd (temporary).

Voluntary and involuntary groups: In voluntary group option is available to become a member, e.g. a football club. A family is an example of involuntary group.

Table 5.1: Differences between primary and secondary social group

	Primary group	*Secondary group*
Physical proximity	Close 'Face to face' contact	Lack of 'Face to face' contact
Social aim	Similar	Not similar
Relationship	'End in itself'	'Means to an end'
Relationship	Direct and personal	Indirect and impersonal
Relationship	Natural and spontaneous	Not natural, specifically developed
Socialization	More important for socialization	Less important for socialization
Social control	Exerts more social control	Exerts limited social control
Function	Makes a human out of an individual	Makes an individual out of humanity
Example	Family is best example of primary social group	Manchester football club is an example of secondary social group

Vertical and horizontal groups: Horizontal group has members belonging to same stratum, e.g. laborers constructing a road, while vertical group has members belonging to different social strata for example a religious section.

Formal and informal groups: Formal groups have legal and formal authority, relatively permanent organization and structure. Informal group do not have legal or formal authority, and do not have hierarchical organization. Playgroup is an example of informal group.

In and out groups: We have a sense of belonging, loyalty and 'We' feeling towards 'In' group. However, 'Out' group are the ones, we feel a sense of indifference, dislike or even hatredness, and 'They' feeling. The basis of In and Out group may be religion, language, social status, etc.

Primary group

Characteristics of primary group

i. Physical Proximity. 'Face to Face' contact.
ii. Identity of Ends. Its members have same social aims.
iii. Relationship is an 'End in Itself'. In primary group, relationship is not a *Means to an End*, but an *End in Itself*.
iv. The relationship between members is personal and direct.
v. The relationship is natural and spontaneous.
vi. Primary social groups exert a powerful influence on social behavior and conduct of its members.

Functions of primary social group

i. Primary group is the nursery of human nature. From it originates the human virtues of love, sympathy, loyalty, cooperation, fair play, sharing, etc.
ii. Primary groups are agencies of socialization, and through them culture is mainly transmitted horizontally, and vertically from one generation to the next.

iii. Primary group satisfies a vital social need of humans, i.e. need for intimate relationship with other humans beings, described as *Man is a social animal.*
iv. Primary social group serves as a powerful instruments of social control.

Secondary group

Characteristics of secondary group

i. Lack of physical proximity or 'Face to Face' contact.
ii. Members do not have common social aim. They are members of the group for a common interest. Secondary relationships are contractual in nature. Hence the relationship is not spontaneous and natural.
iii. The status in secondary groups is identified by functional role played by the member.
iv. The contact between members is usually indirect.
v. The relationship is impersonal.
vi. The relationship is not 'an end in itself' but 'a means to the end'.

Functions of secondary group

For a modern civilization demanding specialization, economic development and competitiveness, secondary groups that have structured organization, well defined functions and responsibilities and formal/legal control are as important as primary groups. These groups provide an individual to fulfill his aspirations, and achieve goals as per his capabilities, thus fulfilling a need of human being, i.e. to achieve excellence in field(s) of his choice.

Collective Behavior

chapter 6

The term collective behavior is now used to refer to crowd, mob and social movements etc.

Crowd

Crowd is defined as collection of considerable number of individuals within a limited space, and responding to some common object of attention. Mere aggregation of people in a limited space is not a crowd, unless there is a common stimulus, and the individuals react to the stimulus in almost similar way.

Characteristics of a crowd

1. Close contact often referred as shoulder to shoulder contact
2. Temporary
3. Unorganized
4. Common interest
5. Anonymity
6. Almost similar reaction, e.g. people in a crowd applaud together
7. The crowd may be 'casual' (e.g. people may assemble when there is a quarrel on road) or 'scheduled' when time, place, speaker and subject are already known to the individuals, e.g. a political rally.
8. Table 6.1 highlights differences between social groups and crowd.

Table 6.1: Crowd vs social group

Social group	*Crowd*
Interaction-direct or indirect	No interaction. Anonymity is important aspect of crowd
Conscious of belonging to the group	Not so
Organized	Unorganized
Permanent	Temporary

Mob

Mob is also a collection of individuals, but here, the individuals are emotionally charged. There may be one or more persons who may perform the role of leader(s). The mob often has a slogan or a symbol, e.g. a flag. The main characteristics of a mob are:

1. **Mental homogeneity:** Members of a mob tend to have a similar feeling, thought and action, although they differ in their education, occupation or intelligence.
2. **Emotionally charged:** High emotional state, e.g. anger, joy, fear, etc. is an important feature of mob.
3. **Sense of anonymity and power:** The behavior of members of the mob is because of feeling of anonymity and sense of Power. They indulge in damage or even killing a person because of high emotional state coupled with sense of power. These two factors are also responsible for decreased sense of responsibility of a mob.

   Table 6.2 highlights similarities and differences between crowd and mob.

Table 6.2: Crowd versus mob

Crowd (Audience)	*Mob*
Temporary collection	Temporary collection
Anonymity	Anonymity
Relatively passive	Active. Even aggressive
Do not have sense of power	Sense of power present
Behavior rational	Behavior irrational
Emotionally not charged	Emotionally highly charged
No leader. All members of the crowd may not consider the speaker their leader	One or more persons may take the role of leader
Slogan or symbol, e.g. flag etc. not present	The mob may start slogan shouting or may have a symbol, e.g. a flag
Not destructive	Usually destructive, but not necessary
May convert into a mob, if speaker infuses high emotions	Does not convert into audience
Usually lawful	Often indulges into unlawful activities
Example: Collection of people watching a street play	Collection of people on the road after a road accident start burning the involved vehicle and beating the driver (unlawful behavior). Here the mob may even burn other vehicles on the road and damage shops that have nothing to do with the accident (irrational behavior)

Public

A dispersed group (unlike crowd), larger membership than crowd. Anonymity is not a feature of Public, hence behavior in not irrational. Individuals in public express and share their experiences about an issue, thus contribute to generate public opinion. Crowd is an acting group while public is a thinking group.

Rumor: It is a collective process in which a communication is passed from person to person, usually by word of mouth, without reference to secure standards of evidence. It causes mutual orientation that makes collective activity possible.

Panic: It is uncoordinated and irrational response to fear. People running out of a building on fire.

Fashion: Collective behavior in matters like dress, house or personal decoration, manner of speech, music, literature, etc. that are current and socially approved. Fashion is subject to change.

Fads: More limited in age group or social stratum. Fads have shorter life than fashions.

Social movement: A social movement represents a collective action to change status quo which the people consider unsatisfactory and to create a new social order.

Leadership is ability to determine the behavior of others in accord with one's wishes.

1. Leadership is a form of dominance.
2. There is super-ordination by leader over his followers.
3. Types- Democratic, Autocratic (dictatorship), Charismatic (religious).

Family

chapter 7

Definition

The family is a group defined by a relationship sufficiently precise and enduring to provide for the procreation and up-bringing of children.

Family is also defined as a group of persons who are related by kinship ties, i.e. relation of blood, marriage or adoption.

Essential characteristics of family

a. The family is composed of persons united by ties of marriage, blood or adoption.
b. **Permanent relation:** Family is a primary social group. The relations are permanent.
c. **Common habitation, home or household:** Even if some members live outside, they consider their household as home.
d. **Nomenclature:** Distinct nomenclature that identifies a family.
e. Family is the fundamental unit of human society.
f. Family is first and most important agency of socialization of children. It is in family we learn qualities as love, sincerity, realizing our responsibilities, etc.

   Family is a very important agency of Social Control.

Functions of family

a. **Procreation:** One of the most important functions of the family is to provide legitimate and responsible basis for procreation.
b. **Childbearing:** Human baby is physically, mentally and socially helpless. For several years after birth, children need the care of adults for development, health and survival. The family plays the role of providing food, clothing and shelter to their offspring. Family is the prime protector and nurturer of the children.
c. **Socialization:** The family is the first and the most important unit for socialization of children. We learn our customs, values, norms, folk ways, habits, behavior, religion and mother tongue in family. Although in later life some of these are modified or changed, but still family remains the most important agency for socialization of humans. It is rightly said that home is the first school and mother, the first teacher.
d. **Educative role:**
    a. In nonliterate societies, the young learn their knowledge as well as skills of their trade in family.
    b. Introduction of school system has not decreased the responsibility of parents in educative role of their children. Parents are expected to do their best to guide, encourage, and support their children through schools and colleges.
e. **Economic functions**
    a. Division of labor. Work is divided among members of the family, as per status and role
    b. Generation of income for household
    c. Organization and care of property. Holding and transmission of property from one generation to the next.

f. **Recreational function:** In preindustrial societies, most of the leisure time was spent with family (except community ceremonies). Even today, family remains a recreational unit, although the role has been modified with increasing role of outside agencies and electronic media as sources of recreation.
g. **Psychological support:** Family is the most important primary group that gives moral and emotional support to its members. It provides defense against social isolation, and loneliness. We receive love, affection, security, protection, mental strength, help and devotion within our family.
h. **Religious functions:** Family life is considered as religious duty of a man and woman. Marriage, procreation and looking after the parents and children is a duty prescribed to us by our religion.
i. **Cultural function:** Family keeps the culture of society alive. Family is the first and the most important agency for vertical and horizontal transmission of culture.

Types of family

Basis of descent

a. **Patriarchal family:** Male head of the family posses all powers. He is owner, administrator and holder of the property. All members of the family are his subordinates.
b. **Matriarchal family:** Woman heads the family. Holds power and property.

Basis of residence

a. **Patrilocal:** Bride and groom live with parents of the groom.
b. **Matrilocal:** Bride and groom live with bride's parents.

Basis of marriage

a. **Monogamous:** One Male: one wife.

b. **Polygamous:** One Male has more than one wives.
c. **Polyandrous:** One wife, more than one husbands.

Based on structure

a. **Joint:** Consists of several nuclear families, joined by kinship relationship (three or more generations) living together in same household, street or locality. It may consist of grandparents, brothers and their spouses and children, sisters with their families, uncles, aunts, nephews and niece (Table 7.1).
b. **Nuclear:** It consists of two married adults (husband and wife) living together in a household with their own or adopted children (till the children are dependent).

Basis of experience

a. **Family of orientation:** The family we are born.
b. **Family of procreation:** After marriage, the individuals enter into family of procreation.

Role of family

In health

a. **Procreation:** Some diseases are transmitted in families. The chances of suffering from these diseases increase when marriages are held among close relatives. This may be the reason why consanguineous marriages (marriages among close relatives) are prohibited.
b. **Childbearing:** Human baby is physically, mentally and socially helpless. For several years after birth, children need the care of adults for development, health and survival. The family has to provide food, clothing and shelter to their offspring. Family is the prime protector and nurturer of children.

Table 7.1: Differences between nuclear and joint family

Nuclear family	*Joint family*
Smaller in size	Larger in size
Status of women is higher. More freedom to take up a job	Status and freedom of women are lower
Husband-wife relationship is more intimate	Less intimate
Husband or wife or both are holders of the property	Property is held jointly by the family, and not by an individual
Family plays less role in social control	Family plays more role in social control
Suits modern life style	Suits traditional life style
Illness disrupts the life of family more	As there are many persons to look after the sick, the life of family is not disrupted to that extent
Nuclear families are more common in urban area	More common in rural areas and towns
Looking after old/ handicapped is more problematic	Less problematic, as some members are always available
Income is not shared	Total income of earning members is pooled

c. **Personal hygiene:** Habits like oral hygiene, bathing, washing of hands before cooking/eating, hygiene during menstruation, care of hair, etc. are learnt at home in family. Many of these remain unchanged throughout life.
d. **Personality development:** The capacity of an individual to withstand stress and strain, and the way he interacts with other persons and different situations are to large extent determined by his experiences in the family.

e. **Education:** In recent years, role of education especially the education of mother (female education) has been recognized as one of the most important factor in health of the family. Hence, education received by child in home, and later in school/college (that is guided and supported by family) is very important for health of the individual and his family.
f. **Mental health:** Family is the most important primary group that gives moral and emotional support to its members. It provides defense against social isolation, and loneliness. We receive love, affection, security, protection, mental strength, help and devotion within our family.
g. **Nutrition:** Family provides nutrition to its members. In addition, it teaches us healthy food habits. It is now being realized that our traditional foods are more nutritious than fast foods like pizza, burgers, colas, etc. that are getting popular in our country due to advertisements.
h. **Environmental Sanitation:** In homes, cleanliness is the way of life. Women of the house, keep their houses clean and presentable. This prevents spread of diseases within members of the family.
i. **Family planning:** Adoption of family welfare measures is a decision to be taken by couples.
h. **Prevention of disease:** Immunization, breastfeeding, weaning food, burning of neem leaves when child is suffering from measles/chickenpox, etc. are actions taken by family for prevention of diseases.

In disease

a. **Care of sick and injured:** Care of sick and injured is an important role that members of family especially mother perform when someone in family falls sick or gets injured. In addition to duties of mother, she performs the duties of nurse. Other members, as per their roles, take the ill person to hospital, look after his diet, personal cleanliness, and provide emotional support.

b. **Care of women during pregnancy and childbirth:** Pregnancy is a physiological state, but requires special management. Family members have to look after the diet, share duties, provide psychological support and also ensure regular antenatal checkups, prepare for the delivery (at home or in hospital) and also for the arrival of the newborn. In our culture, there are many customs related with pregnancy and child birth. In some communities, the first delivery is conducted at home the parents the girl, so that she is better looked after by her mother. Similarly forty days of restriction on outdoor movement of the mother after delivery ensures her recovery and also prevent infection to her and new born.
c. **Care of elderly:** In old age, individuals suffer from diseases of almost all systems. Their motor activity, sensory organs and mental faculties start declining. They also suffer from diseases like diabetes, hypertension, cancers etc. These diseases require continuous medical care which is costly. On the other hand, in old age one is incapable of earning. So he is dependent on family for his needs. In our culture, the children have to look after their old parents, for all their needs.
d. **Care of handicapped:** Presence of a physically or mentally handicapped person is a challenge to any family. Where as a sick person is likely to recover after few days, a handicapped person may require life time support. This poses a continuous physical, social, psychological and economic stress on the family.
e. **Examples of effect on health**
    a. **Broken family:** A broken family is one where parents have separated, or death has occurred of one or both parents. It has been seen that the children who are

victims of broken family are more prone to deviant behavior and personality disorders.

b. **Problem family:** Problem families are those in which home life is utterly un-satisfactory. It may be due to extreme poverty, mental illnesses, marital disharmony, character defects, alcoholism, drug addiction etc. Children who are reared in such environment often become victim of prostitution, drug addiction, criminals, beggary etc.
c. **Poor environment condition:** For example, poor standards of sanitation in the house, poor standards of nutrition due to poverty or lack of knowledge, unhealthy customs (e.g. purdhah custom) etc. are associated with higher rates of diseases among family members.
d. **Education status especially of mother:** Higher the education of mother (lady of the house) better is the health of the family. All indicators of health are better in Kerala, as compared to other States, just because of better educational status of population especially females, although the economic status is better in many other states, e.g. Punjab.

Effect of illness on family

a. **Economic burden:** Any disease, even a mild one like common cold or diarrhea causes expenditure. In serious and prolonged diseases, the expenditure runs into thousands. This comes as an economic burden on the family, disrupting its economic planning. Poor people may fall into debt-trap on such occasions.
b. **Disturbance in routine activities of the family:** Any illness disturbs the routine of the family. The members of the family may not go to office/school due to illness. Someone may have to stay awake at night to look after the patient. If

admitted in the hospital, routine of many family members get disturbed.

c. **Leisure time:** Leisure time of all members gets disturbed. Recreational activities may have to be cancelled or postponed due to illness.

d. **Psychological stress:** It is natural for patient to be irritable, anxious, depressed etc. due to the pain and discomfort caused by illness. However, other members also get psychological stressed due to illness in the family. Lack of sleep, rest, extra work, financial burden, anxiety, etc. makes everyone stressed. In such situation, sharing of responsibility, mutual understanding especially between husband and wife go a long way in facing the challenge. The situation is getting more and more challenging with nuclear families and with working women.

e. **Social stigma:** Some diseases, e.g. AIDS, leprosy, etc. are associated with considerable social stigma in our society. Families may be socially boycotted or avoided, if there is a case of such diseases in the family.

Socialization

chapter

8

What do we understand by socialization? Unlike animals, whose behavior is mostly instinctive (based on instincts), humans have to learn appropriate ways of behavior during our life time. It is said that 'we are not born human, but we become human during the course of our life, by interacting with other human beings. Our humanness is thus, a totally social product. This process by which humans learn to become members of the society, by learning the norms and values of the society, and also learning his social roles (as son, brother, student, neighbor, friend, parents, teacher, physiotherapist, etc.) is called socialization.

Features or characteristics of socialization

a. Learning process by which we learn norms and values of society
b. Also learn ways to perform our social role
c. Socialization occurs mainly in childhood, but the process continues through out life. A sixty-years-old person is also learning social role of Grandpa.
d. Two way process. Child learns from her parents, at the same time the parents are learning bringing up child.
e. Through socialization, society transmits its culture from one generation to next generation.
f. Socialization is important for personality development of individuals.

Role of socialization

The process of socialization has a dual role, one concerning the growth of an individual, the other concerning the society, of which the individual as a member. It is also viewed as a process by which society creates persons suitable to carry out its functional requirements.

Types of socialization

Primary socialization

a. Refers to socialization in early life-childhood.
b. Occurs mainly at home.
c. Primary social groups i.e. family, peer group and neighborhood are main agencies for primary socialization.
d. **Informal:** No special agency for imparting primary socialization (unlike secondary socialization).
e. Occurs naturally during growth of the child.
f. By close contact (face to face relationship)
g. Intimacy, prolonged contact and affection promote transmission from parents/elders to child.
h. The child also wants to gain approval of parents, elders by copying their behavior.
i. Language (mother tongue), the most important aspect of personality is learnt thorough primary socialization.
j. By five years of age, 'peer group' also starts playing its role in socialization. Rules of friendship, games etc are learnt between friends.
k. Although secondary socialization becomes more important in our adult life, primary socialization through family, peer groups and neighborhood continues throughout life.

Secondary socialization

a. Refers to socialization in adult life. Occurs mainly at educational institutes, workplace, etc. (outside home).

b. Secondary social groups are main agencies for secondary socialization.
c. Formal. Special agencies e.g. schools, media (radio, TV, face book, newspapers) etc. assist secondary socialization.
d. Not by face to face relationship
e. Intelligence, desire to improve personality, achieve his personal aspirations promote learning. For example, we learn American way of life, e.g. (pronunciation) for settling in US.

Important differences between primary and secondary socialization are mentioned in Table 8.1.

Table 8.1 : Differences between primary and secondary socialization

	Primary socialization	*Secondary socialization*
Time period	Mainly in childhood	During adult life
Done mainly by	Primary social groups	Secondary social groups
Place	Mainly at home and neighborhood	At schools, colleges, workplace (away from home and neibhorhood
Agency	No formal agency	Special agencies like educational institutes, media, workplaces
Type	Informal	Formal
Contact	Close (Face to face)	Not 'Face to face'
Motivating factor	Love, friendship, approval of parents and peer group	To 'do well' in life
Example	Mother tongue is learnt through primary socialization	Other languages say English is learnt through secondary socialization

Agencies of socialization

Family

a. First agency
b. Most important agency
c. Informal
d. Language (mother tongue) is learnt at home.
e. Intimacy, prolonged contact and affection promote transmission from parents/elders to child.
f. The child also wants to gain approval of parents, elders by copying their behavior
g. Two way socialization
h. In contemporary society role of family is gradually decreasing. Children nowadays do not, unquestionably, adopt the attitudes and outlook of their parents
i. Sex related issues are not discussed in our homes. Hence the adolescence learns it from his peers who may not themselves have correct information.
j. Stress in family (broken, problem families) seriously affects the personality and behavior of child who may develop deviant behavior.

Peer group

i. Peer group means friendship group of same age.
ii. Child over 4 to 5 years of age starts spending considerable time with his friends.
iii. Peer group are formed in schools, colleges and at work places.
iv. In 'peer group' parental control is not present, child/ adolescent/adult feels more free and relaxed. This mental state promotes learning especially rules of games, friendship, cooperation, fashion, fads, subjects that are taboo at home, e.g. sex.

Educational institutes

Educational Institutes from kindergarten to universities are important agencies of socialization. Although the socialization process has already begun at home, but education system remains one of the pillars where socialization is not only transmitted but also refined. Education system remains central by which the society consciously sets out to transmit norms and values to next generation. School curricula e.g. text books on history, geography, languages, science, etc. are meant to inculcate norms and attitudes that the society considers appropriate for its next generation.

Mass media

The mass media i.e. TV, newspapers, periodicals, radio and films are important socializing agents. The media communicate social attitudes, norms, public opinion, opinions of specialists on issues. Advertisements also help socialization. Of all the mass media, TV has emerged as the most powerful. TV is influencing the behavior, attitudes, values and norms of not even adults, but also of children. TV has been blamed for declining moral values in society. It is influencing diet pattern (promoting high calorie fast food like pizzas, burgers, chips, colas etc.), fashion as well as fads. Film stars, soap opera artists, National talent search shows, comedy shows, etc. have produced new ideals who are imitated by young as well as not so young.

Religion

Religion exerts powerful influence on man's behavior. Not speaking lies or ill of others, not stealing, cheating or being unfaithful in marriage, diet (veg), benevolence, etc. are often directed by our religious faith or fear of God. Religion also has negative effects, e.g. it promotes exploitation, idleness, untouchability, communalism, etc.

Others

a. Voluntary organizations
b. Social clubs
c. Caste groups

To conclude, socialization is a life long learning process, which occurs through number of agencies. Of these, family is generally believed to be the most important. But it should not imply that attitudes and values acquired in childhood are not open to significant changes throughout individual's life cycle.

Social Control

chapter
9

Social Control is defined as "the system of devices whereby the society brings its members into conformity with the accepted standards of behavior".

Another definition: It is a process by which the individual is made group responsive; and by which social organization is built and maintained".

Main features of social control

i. Social control is an influence.
ii. The influence is exercised by the society.
iii. The influence is exercised for promoting the welfare of the society.

Need for social control

i. Maintain social order
ii. To regulate or control behavior of individuals
iii. To maintain social unity
iv. To support social sanctions those are applied to enforce when an individual deviates from prescribed behavior.
v. **Social change and social control:** As the function of social control is to protect and perpetuate the existing social system, it tends to resist social change.

Means (agencies) of social control

Informal	*Formal*
Beliefs	Law
Ideals and Ideologies	Education
Folkways	Punishments
Mores	
Customs	
Religion	
Art and literature	
Humor and satire	
Public opinion	

Informal means of social control

Informal means of social control are called informal because they are part of socialization process. There is no special agency to enforce them. Primary social groups are the most important means of social control.

a. **Beliefs:** It is a conviction that a particular thing is true. It may be true or false, but we are convinced that it is true. For example, God, hell, heaven.
b. **Ideals and ideologies:** From childhood, the society through various means tries to project the Great persons like Mahatma Gandhi, Lord Buddha, Ram, and Guru Nanak, etc. Their monuments are made, pictures are placed in schools, and quotes by them are written in schools/projected on media. Similarly ideologies like Gandhism, Leninism, capitalism, communism, etc. are taught to us.
c. **Folkways:** Folkways are accepted ways of behaviour in a society. Social life is full of challenges, and man seems to have various ways of dealing with them. The 'way' found the best for a given challenge is accepted by the group (folk) as accepted way of behavior, hence the term 'folkways'.

Folkways are passed to succeeding generations, but new elements are added based on changing needs of time. Folkways are subtle means of social control. It is rightly said that no member of a community ever questions a folkway, nor there is ever a need to enforce a folkway.

d. **Mores:** Mores are customs that are considered to be of great significance, and rather indispensable to welfare of society. Unlike Folkways, Mores are more deeply rooted in society and change less frequently. Reaction to non-conformity of Mores is stronger, hence Mores are stronger means of social control than Folkways.

   Table 4.1 further clarifies the differences between Folkways and Mores.

e. **Customs:**
   1. Include Folkways and Mores.
   2. Customs persist for long time, often from one generation to next.
   3. Unlike law, there is no specific authority to declare, prescribe or enforce them.
   4. Accepted by society
   5. We follow them because they have been accepted in past
   6. Customs compel individuals to conform to accepted standard behavior, and control selfish impulses.
   7. Important means of social control
   8. The importance of customs as means of social control is decreasing due to modernization.

f. **Religion:** Religion is an important source of social control. For many individuals it is more powerful than law. It influences behavior. It also forms basis of many mores and customs. It also promotes charity, benevolence, truthfulness and faithfulness.

g. **Humor and satire:** Cartoons, satire on TV

h. **Public opinion:** Important means of control of politicians, leaders, institutions, policies as well as individuals.

i. **Art and literature:** Scripture, moral value of a story is often discussed in classes. Music, dance, drama, etc. also influence human behavior.

Formal means of social control

Law

a. Most important formal means of social control.
b. Primitive societies are controlled by informal means, but as the societies grow in size and complexities, rules and regulations are enforced which define the necessary conduct by individuals. The law also specifies the penalties that will be imposed on violation.
c. Law is enacted by agencies authorized to do so (legislative role). It's enforcement is also entrusted to specific agencies (executive role, e.g. traffic police). The individual or group of individuals violating the law is punished by another agency (judicial role).
d. Laws lay down rules regulating driving (left side of road), Hindu Marriage Act 1955, provides social security (ESI Act), ensures transparency (RTI Act), protects health (Prevention of Food Adulteration Act) and also prohibits untouchability, taking/giving bribes and smoking in public places.

These are few examples of law controlling behavior of individuals and group of individuals for the welfare of society.

Table 9.1 highlights the differences between Mores and Law.

Education

a. Education is as important as law, as formal means of social control.
b. Education is also a means of correcting wrong/bad habits or attitudes learnt by the child at his home.
c. We see that many laws, e.g. Dowry act is not being followed by society. People are still smoking in public places. Thus enactment of a law is not an end it itself. Hence, education

Table 9.1: Differences between Mores and Law

Mores	*Law*
Mores are pattern of behavior that are regulated by the society	Law is related to pattern of behavior enforced by the State.
Nonconformity to Mores is punished by society (e.g. social boycott)	Nonconformity to law is called crime, and is punishable by State (fines, jail, etc.)
All Mores are not laws. Example 'purdah' system is one of the Mores, but law does not enforce it	Some laws may not be accepted by society. For example, child marriage, dowry, untouchability, etc. are forbidden by law, but still prevalent in our society

plays an important part, and attempts to bring about changes in knowledge, attitudes and practices that are conducive to health of populations and welfare of the society.

Punishment

Punishment refers to an action or actions taken by an authority (individual, e.g. class teacher, institution like Nursing Council of India or state like police) after a behavior (e.g. copying, negligence in nursing care of a patient or financial fraud), and aims to eliminate or at least reduce the likelihood that behavior will be repeated in future. It has been found that punishments are more effective if they are given at the earliest after an unwarranted behavior, and are repeated every single time the behavior is repeated. In practice, both these conditions are not met in most of the societies, thus making punishments less effective. Punishments (e.g. spanking of children by parents) are also responsible for antisocial and aggressive behavior by the recipient, more so if the punished feels that she/he has not been guilty or is being discriminated.

Social Stratification

chapter
10

Social stratification is one of the most important characteristics of societies. Inequality in societies due to age, physical or mental ability is natural. However, the inequalities that are created by individuals in society are called social stratification. Another characteristic of social stratification is its rather permanent nature.

Definition

It is horizontal division of society in permanent groups or categories linked with each other by the relationship of superiority and subordination.

The higher strata enjoy following advantages:

a. Better quality of life
b. Higher social status
c. More political influence
d. In addition, though not necessarily so, the higher strata are also financially better than lower strata.

Examples of social stratification

a. Slavery
b. Caste system in Hinduism
c. Social class.

Open and closed system

Open system

When individuals can change their status with relatively ease, the system is called open system. Social Class is an example of open system.

Closed system

In closed system it is not possible to change the status. The status is decided at birth. Hindu caste system is examples of closed system.

Social mobility

By social mobility is meant movement of persons and groups up or down the ranking order of a social stratification system.

Types of mobility

a. **Horizontal:** Here the person moves in the same stratum, e.g. a nurse changing job from one hospital to another.
b. **Vertical:** Movement of an individual from one social stratum to another, example a peon son becoming President of India.

Factors favoring social mobility

a. Modern society
b. Urbanization
c. Industrialization
d. Better communication facilities
e. Educational opportunities
f. Marriages
g. Welfare policies of the state, e.g. Reservation for SCs/STs
h. Change of religion, e.g. many low caste Hindus are converting to Christianity to come out of low social status.

Obstacles to social mobility

a. Resistance of society, e.g. caste system
b. Religious sanction, e.g. caste system
c. Corruption

In our context, social mobility is not possible in caste system, meaning it is a closed system. In class (upper, middle, lower classes) social mobility is possible, hence it is an open system.

Important basis for social stratification

a. Age
b. Gender
c. Birth-caste system
d. Race—Whites versus blacks in US
e. Religion
f. Political
g. Class usually based on occupation, income and education.

Caste system in India

Origin of caste system

Traditional explanation: Divine in origin. The 'Rig Veda' mentions that the four Varna emerged from different parts of *Purusha*, Brahmans from Mouth, Kshatriyas from arms; Vaishyas from thighs; and Shudras from feet.

Racial Theory: Aryan versus Dravidians. Aryan placed themselves superior to Dravidians, who were defeated and called Dasus or inferior. This theory gave importance to physical features and fairer color in stratification of the Indian society.

Occupational theory: Nesfield proposed that division of labor was the basis for origin of castes. As manual craftsmanship was best learnt from childhood onwards, the caste system became inter-generational.

Political theory: Caste system was devised and strengthened by Brahmins to enjoy exclusive privileges. Priests through rituals and ceremonies could impose restrictions over others to preserve their superiority and authority over others.

Caste system

Varna and caste: In Vedic period (1500-800 BC) the society was divided into four groups or Varnas-Brahmans (priests, knowledge-men); Kshatriyas (warriors); Vaishyas (traders) and Shudras (workmen). The Varnas were based on 'Gunas' and these groups were not totally closed; Individuals could move from one Varna to another and inter-Varnas marriages were permitted. Four varnas were not caste. Caste or jatis developed in late Vedic period, based on occupation. Over period of time 'Jatis' grew in numbers. The Varnas are four while there are about 2,500 Jatis in modern India. There are hundred of jatis in each Varna. Most Indian scholars believe that Varna system and caste system are two different systems that coexisted for at least 1,000 years. The hierarchy in Varnas is well laid, while in Jatis it is more ambiguous.

Important features of caste system

a. **Birth:** Caste decided by birth. Unalterable.
b. Hierarchical division of society.
c. Restriction of sharing of food, drinks and social interaction. Food especially cooked food is not accepted by higher caste. Wells were separate. Social interaction is prohibited, although occupational interactions are not.
d. **Restriction on privileges and religious restrictions:** Untouchables lived separately, and forbidden to enter temples and draw water from same wells. It was believed that physical contact (touching) causes pollution (Impurity).
e. Restrictions on choice of occupation

f. **Restriction of marriages:** Caste is an endogamous group. Inter caste marriages were declared null and void.

Changing caste system

Indian caste system has not only withstood the time, but also opposition by Buddhism, Jainism, Islam, Christianity, and Sikhism. Many reform movements like Arya Samaj, Brahma Samaj, Bhakti Movement RamaKrishna Mission, etc. tried to denounce the caste system declaring that it had no religious sanction. Mahatma Gandhi struggled hard to eradicate the evil of untouchablility in India.

Vedic period: Four Varnas. The stratification was open.

Post vedic period: Jatis started to develop and strengthen.

Pre-British period: In pre-British period, although individuals could not change their Caste, but some Jatis succeeded in raising their status. This became possible when, by circumstances or prolonged efforts, the lower caste as group improved its economic position. Many royal families came from Shudras. In Moghul period many Kayasthas, who by occupation were 'record writers' rose high in public life, wealth and education because of close association with Political power.

British period: British rulers introduced several laws in order to bringout about fundamental changes in traditional caste system. Western type of education, equality in matters of administration, increasing opportunities of employment, better transportation facilities, industrialization, etc. indirectly diluted the rigidity of caste system. Social reform movements like Arya Samaj and Brahma Samaj attempted to ward off traditional caste system. In spite of all these, the major social units remained the same. Opportunities were more available to higher caste because of their head start in education and economic arenas.

Post independence period: The traditional caste system has been profoundly altered after independence. On 26 January 1950, Indian Constitution proclaimed India as sovereign Democratic Republic with aim of casteless and classless society. The constitution provides the fundamental right of equality to all citizens irrespective of caste, creed and religion. Following factors have played important role:

a. **Democratic system.** Power has rapidly passed into lower caste. Tamil Nadu, UP, and Bihar are examples where lower caste CMs have run the state for long periods.
b. Industrialization and urbanization.
c. Increased occupational mobility.
d. Educational opportunities.
e. Land reforms.
f. Reservations for lower castes in education, jobs, electoral seats.
g. Modern Indian society emphasizes competition, individual achieve-ment and equality of opportunity.
h. Role of media.
i. Better communication systems.

Is the caste system dying?

1. In rural India the caste system still exists and shows no sign of dying. In villages, the dominant caste (not necessarily the upper caste), by virtue of their control of land and capital enjoy power and influence. The landless laborers and lower castes remain powerless, dependent on land owners for employment and help at the time of distress. Millions live in debt bondage.
2. The caste division has now become an important political card, and many political parties are dependent upon caste division for vote banks.
3. Reservation policy itself is fueling caste consciousness.

4. Endogamy is formidable pillar which still supports caste division.

Social class

Another system of social stratification is social class. This system gets more important as the society modernizes. Social class is determined by economic status, level of education, occupation, life style etc. It also has direct health implications as it is related with the availability of health resources and their utilization.

Social scientists have often use occupation as parameter to determine social class of an individual. The advantages of using occupation are:

1. Related with education
2. Related with income
3. Related with status
4. Related with values and life style
5. Related with obligations to society.

Occupational classification

- I. Professional occupation
- II. Intermediate occupation
- III. N. Non manual skilled worker
- III. M. Manual skilled worker
- IV. Partly skilled worker
- V. Unskilled worker.

However, purchasing power (income) and education also are important criteria to describe role, obligations and status of an individual. Hence social classes are now best described using scales that integrate occupation, income and education in defining social class. These scales are called socioeconomic scales. Many scales have been developed for use in developed and developing nations, and for rural and urban communities.

Kuppuswamy's socioeconomic scale is often used in medicosocial research in India. It is based on:

i. **Education:** Divided into seven subgroups. Score 1 to 7
ii. **Occupation:** Divided into seven sub groups. Score 1 to 10.
iii. **Family income per month:** Divided into seven subgroups. Score 1 to 12.

Kuppuswamy's socioeconomic class

Score	*Class*
26-29	Upper (I)
16-25	Upper Middle (II)
11-15	Lower Middle (III)
5-10	Upper Lower (IV)
< 5	Lower (V)

Important differences between caste and class systems of social stratification are mentioned in Table 10.1

Table 10.1: Difference between caste and class

Caste	*Class*
By birth	Not by birth. achieved in life
Closed system	Open system
Believed to have divine sanction, hence supported by religion	Secular in nature, not endorsed by religion
Endogamous, marriages outside caste not permitted	Interclass marriages are permitted
Relative status of caste stratification is well established	Relative status in class in not fixed. Presently financial power has overtaken education and occupation
Caste consciousness is not important feature of caste system	Class consciousness is present

Social class and health

Large number of studies has linked social class to incidence of diseases. Income, occupation and education are important determinants of health. In general:

1. Communicable ciseases have higher incidence in lower classes.
2. Infant, child and maternal mortality rates decrease as we move from lower class to upper class.
3. However, in India the incidence of non-communicable diseases of hypertension, diabetes, coronary artery diseases are higher in Social class I than in other classes. This is because of rapidly changing life style of individuals in this class.
4. The utilization of health services is better in Upper social classes. Family welfare services, immunization, number of consultations of doctor, antenatal, institutional delivery and postnatal care are utilized more by upper classes than lower.

Factors responsible for health differences among social classes

i. **Physical environment:** Upper classes enjoy better physical environ-ment e.g. safe water, housing, disposal of wastes.
ii. **Nutrition:** Nutrition is an important determinant of health. Balanced diet with adequate amount of proteins, vitamins and minerals ensure better immunity in individuals belonging to upper classes. However, overeating and more consumption of junk food, and sedentary life style are responsible for higher rates of life style diseases e.g diabetes, hypertension etc. in upper classes.
iii. **Availability of medical facilities:** Urban centric distribution of medical resources.
iv. **Educational status.**
v. **Economic status.**
vi. **Attitude towards health and disease.**

Social Change

chapter 11

It is rightly said that change is the only thing that is constant in this world. All societies are undergoing change. MacIver and Page has said that "Society is becoming, not a being. It is a process, not a product".

Definition: Social change has been defined as alterations or modifications in structure and functioning of society over a period of time.

Main characteristics of social change

i. Social change is a universal phenomenon. All societies are changing all the times.
ii. Social change affects the whole community (not an individual).
iii. The speed of social change varies in different periods.
iv. Definite prediction of social change is not possible.
v. Social change is a chain reaction.
vi. Main changes are either modification or replacement.
vii. Social change occurs due to interactions of multiple factors.

Social change and cultural change

Cultural changes denote change in norms, values and beliefs of a given society, while social change means changes in social structure and social behavior. Although the two are different, but both are closely inter woven, as social structure and human behavior are guided by social values, norms and beliefs.

Social progress

Progress means change in the right direction. Progress should include improvements both materially and morally. As any social change is considered by some as beneficial, and by others as retrograde, sociologists prefer to use the term change over progress.

Opposition to social change

i. Desire for stability
ii. Ignorance
iii. Habits and traditions
iv. Economic costs
v. Vested interest
vi. Intellectual laziness
vii. Social control.

Factors facilitating social change

i. **Demographic factors:** A change in size, composition, density, distribution and migration of populations is considered an important factor for social change.
ii. **Technological factors:** Marx highlighted the role played by technology and inventions in bringing social changes. Industrial revolution is considered as having responsible for (a) Moving people from fields to factories (b) Rural to urban areas (c) Disintegration of joint families (d) Occupational mobility (e) Dominance of urban ways of life (f) Emergence of new classes (g) Increase in specialization (h) Emergence of trade unions (i) Rise of democracy and many other changes. TVs changed the social behavior of whole generation. Today we are witnessing changes in our behavior and ways of life due to mobile phones and internet.
iii. **Cultural diffusion or acculturation:** When people of different culture come into contact with each other,

there occurs diffusion of culture. This process is called acculturation. In this way culture acts as triggering factor for social change.

Theories regarding direction of social change

i. **Deterioration theory:** From perfectness to disaster. Satyug to Kalyug and Maha Pralay.
ii. **Evolutionary theory:** This theory uses Darwin's theory of biological evolution to social change. Societies struggle with one another for survival, and this struggle changes the simple and homogeneous societies towards complex and heterogeneous societies.
iii. **Equilibrium theory:** As per this theory, any change in one element of society, will cause change in other elements to restore balance or equilibrium.
iv. **Cyclic theory:** This theory postulates that the changes in societies are not linear, but cyclic. Societies undergo periods of growth, maturity and decline.

Cultural lag

This concept was first propagated by Professor WF Ogburn. He distinguished between material (e.g. TV, computer, washing machine) and non-material culture (values, beliefs, norms). He proposed that the changes in material culture were rapid, and nonmaterial culture follows the changes in material culture. Thus nonmaterial culture lags behind technological advancement. This is called cultural lag. Many sociologists do not agree with this concept, and say that "Ogburn has made a tail (technology) wagging the dog (culture)".

Social Security

chapter 12

Definition

Security that society furnishes through appropriate organization, against certain risks to which its members are exposed.

The risks usually covered are against are:

i. Sickness
ii. Loss of job
iii. Invalidity
iv. Maternity
v. Old age
vi. Death.

Social security

For general public

i. Insurance for life, disease, crops, etc.
ii. National Rural Employment Guarantee Act, 2005.

For government servants

i. Pension
ii. Gratuity
iii. Family Pension
iv. Insurance
v. Provident Fund
vi. Medical cover
vii. Medical cover for retired.

For industrial workers

i. Workmen's Compensation Act, 1923
ii. Central Maternity Benefit Act, 1961
iii. Employees State Insurance Act, 1948
iv. The Family Pension Scheme, 1971
v. The Factories Act, 1948
vi. The Mines Act, 1952
vii. The Persons with Disabilities (Equal Opportunity, Protection of Rights and Full Participation) Act, 1995.

The Persons with Disabilities (equal opportunity, protection of rights and full participation) Act, 1995

National Sample Survey conducted in 1991 revealed that 1.9% of the total population of India is having one of the following disabilities:

a. Visual disabilities
b. Hearing disabilities
c. Speech disabilities
d. Locomotor disabilities.

On the basis of these findings, and to prevent, treat, support and rehabilitate disabled the Persons with disabilities Act was passed by the Parliament in 1995.

Definition of disability: The Act encompasses following disabilities:

i. Blindness and visually handicapped
ii. Disabilities due to leprosy
iii. Hearing impairment
iv. Locomotor disability
v. Mental retardation
vi. Mental illnesses
vii. Any individual should have 40 percent or more disablement to be included as disabled under the Act.

Objectives of the Act

a. Act provides for preventive as well as promotive aspects of disability
b. Rehabilitation of disabled through education, vocational training and employment.
c. Research and manpower development
d. Creation of barrier free environment
e. Reservation in educational institutes and employment
f. Unemployment allowances
g. Special insurance schemes
h. Establishment of homes.

Organization

i. Central Level Coordination Committee
ii. State Level Coordination Committee
iii. Executive Committee
iv. Functions of these Committees (a) develop policies (b) Coordinate and review activities of Governmental and Non-Governmental Organizations (NGOs) (c) Evaluation of policies and programs for disabled.

Important provisions under the Act

a. Prevention and early detection of disabilities.
b. Screening of children once a year.
c. Actions for prevention and progression of the disabilities.
d. Maternal and child health care
e. Awareness campaigns for public
f. Training of staff of primary health centers to assist in this work
g. Education facilities to the disabled
h. Free education till age of 18 years for every disabled child
i. Three percent of seats reserved for disabled in all educational institution receiving government grants

j. Training of teachers.
k. Employment. Three percent of vacancies in government jobs reserved for disabled.
l. Mass awareness through mass media
m. Nondiscrimination of the disabled
n. Financial aid to NGOs providing assistance to disabled
o. Redressal of grievances.

Miscellaneous Topics

chapter **13**

Religion

Definition

Religion is a system of beliefs, symbols and practices (e.g. rituals) which is based on the idea of the sacred, and which unites the believers into a socio-religious group. Through religion people attempt to cope with the ultimate problems of human life.

Characteristics

Study of all religions of the world reveals that five elements are basic in religion:

a. **Belief in super natural power:** In all religions, is the belief that there are supernatural powers, i.e. power(s) beyond human observable world.
b. **Belief in the holy:** There are certain things in each religion that are considered holy or sacred.
c. **Rituals:** Prayers, bath in Ganges, wearing of special clothes, head shaving, etc. are rituals associated with Hindu religion. Similarly there are rituals associated with every religion.
d. **Acts defined as sinful:** Every religion mentions acts that are prohibited and sinful. These may be acts of commission or omission. Doing or not doing these act brings wrath of Supernatural, and is also creates sense of guilt.
e. Methods of Salvation, *Nirvana*, Heaven, etc. are considered goals of human birth.

Social functions

Social solidarity: Religion by collective obedience reinforces social solidarity among believers of same religions. All religions of the world promote tolerance, patience, truthfulness, honesty, non theft, non adultery, etc. thus tend to bring harmony in the society. However, recent decades have shown us that religion as basic cause of division and disruption of social order. Religion has now become the force behind fundamentalism and terrorism.

Social control: Religion plays an important role in the mechanism of social control. It acts as an agent of social control by providing rewards for good conduct and punishment for bad. Being always seen by the supernatural, we conduct ourselves for the good of the society even when not being observed by other human beings.

Social change: Religion can also act as a catalyst for social change. Protestants concept of 'work ethics' played an important role in growth of new social order of capitalism.

Important religions in the world

a. **Judaism:** Official religion of State of Israel
b. **Christianity:** Began as a sect of Judaism. Largest following. Catholicism, Protestantism, Eastern Orthodoxy are main branches of Christianity.
c. **Islam:** 2nd largest religion in the world
d. Hinduism
e. Buddhism
f. **Confucianism:** Religion of Traditional China. Confucius who lived in 6th Century BC is considered as a teacher (wisest of the wise) and not a god.

Interview

Interview is a method for getting information from living persons through formal contact. Information can be obtained through personal face to face interview, through telephonic/ internet contact or through postal questionnaires.

Objectives

i. Obtain information through face to face association
ii. To study the personality of the individual, his social and psychological background
iii. Interview are also useful as these are two way process. The informant, e.g. job seeker) also wants to know the organization he will be working for.

Types

i. **Structured interview:** In this type, a scheduled is prepared and the interviewer asks the questions as per the schedule only. The interviewer does not have authority to change the language, sequence or type of questions.
ii. **Unstructured interview:** No prepared schedule or questionnaire is available. Here the researcher collects the information by free discussion. The interviewee gives his opinion or reactions on the subject under discussion, while the interviewer guides him by asking relevant or prompting questions. In this type, the interviewer has to be more trained than the structured interviewer to comprehend the responses of the interviewee.
iii. **Depth interviews:** These are used to identify the attitudes, habits, motives, reasons for behavior, etc. of the subject. Here the interviewer wants to identify *whys* behind the choices of the interviewee.

Steps

i. **Establish contact:** Prior appointment, place and time should be fixed. The subject to be discussed in the interview may also be communicated so that the interviewee is mentally prepared for the interview.

ii. **Starting interview:** After introductions, the objectives of interview should be explained in simple understandable language. Confidentiality of information obtained should be assured.
iii. **Interview:** During interview the interviewer should:
    - Establish good rapport.
    - Let the interviewee do most of the talking.
    - Controversial aspects should be avoided or asked at the end.
    - Difficult question, e.g. about addictions, sex, etc. should be asked in the last.
    - If the interviewee gets emotional, time should be given to regain his composure by remaining silent for some time. If necessary, the interviewee memory should be refreshed by pointing out what he was saying last.
    - Probe questions should be asked with care.
    - If the interviewee loses track, he should be brought back on the main issue diplomatically without offending him.
    - Words or gestures of encouragement should be said from time to time.
iv. **Recording:** The writing during interview should be done to the minimum. Audio or video recoding may be done after obtaining permission of the interviewee.
v. **Closing the interview:** The interview should not be closed abruptly.
vi. Report should be compiled at the earliest, when the narration and information is still fresh.

Advantages

i. In interview, the nonresponse can be kept to minimum.
ii. Interviews provide flexibility. Questions can be explained in different ways with examples.

.ompetent interviewer can differentiate between facts ɲd fiction by studying gestures, body language, tone, etc.

Unstructured interviews can provide information regarding opinions, values, attitudes, etc.

ɹisadvantages or limitation

i. More time consuming.
ii. Costly.
iii. Sample size is often small, because of above points.
iv. Structured interview does not provide any flexibility.
v. Interview bias. This bias occurs due to leading questions by interviewer, behavior/accent, etc. of the interviewer. The respondent may try to give answers that he thinks the interviewer wants.

Important points for interviewer

i. Maintain good eye contact.
ii. Give undivided attention. Mobile phones should be on silent mode.
iii. Use language that is understood. Avoid technical words.
iv. Open ended questions are better than closed ended question.
v. If interviewee uses a technical word, clarify its meaning. Word Gastric is used by patients for almost many symptoms of GI Tract.
vi. Facilitate verbally and nonverbally. A touch of hand sometimes encourages the most.
vii. Keep note taking to minimum.

Medicosocial work

Medicosocial work originated during 1895 in England. Now it is an integral part of medicine.

Objectives

- i. To find the social background of disease, thus hel, physician to make 'social diagnosis' and to treat the patient more holistically.
- ii. Utilize community resources for medical, social, vocational and psychological rehabilitation of patient.

Medicosocial worker

- i. Paramedical worker
- ii. Trained in medicosocial work and in art of interviewing people.
- iii. Employed in hospitals, chronic diseases clinics like TB, leprosy, HIV/AIDS, mental health clinics, family planning, etc.
- iv. Medicosocial worker is the link between the hospital/ institution and the community.
- v. Medicosocial worker visits the family and community of the patient.
- vi. He/she studies the personal, social, economic, environmental and cultural factors that are related with the disease.
- vii. MS worker also tries to help the patient through utilization of community resources.
- viii. Thus he plays a vital role in rehabilitation of patient suffering from chronic diseases or disabilities. Social, psychological, vocational and community based medical rehabilitation are more effective when conducted in association with MS worker.

Medicosocial history

Factors Related to Individual

- i. Personal Data. Name, age, gender, address, mobile number

ii. Education
iii. Occupation
iv. Rural/Urban
v. Immunization
vi. Habits—Physical exercise, diet, smoking, alcohol or substance abuse, sexual promiscuity. (sensitive questions should be asked near the end of the interview).
vii. Knowledge, Attitudes and Practices (KAP) regarding common diseases and about disease under study.
viii. Psychological Status (To be observed) cheerful, depressed, anxious
ix. Separation from spouse/ family and reasons there of
x. Social factors in the family.

Type of family

i. Organization of Family. Structure, total members, head of the family
ii. Caste
iii. Education. General level of education in family
iv. Occupation
v. Income
vi. Socioeconomic scale
vii. KAP of family members
viii. Availability, accessibility, affordability, quality and utilization of health services including alternative system of health.
ix. Sources of entertainment in family.
x. Social aberrations in family problem/broken family, single parent family, alcoholism, delinquency, any chronic stress.

Environmental factors in family

i. Housing. General description, ventilation, lighting, overcrowding

ii. Source of water
iii. Sanitary latrine available or not
iv. Food Hygiene. Kitchen, storage of raw and cooked food, fly/ rodent nuisance
v. Nutrition. Assessment of calorie intake, major macro and micro nutrients deficiency.

Psychological factors in family

i. Social aberration or social stress in family
ii. Support the patient is likely to get from family.

Factors in work place

i. Details of work—any occupational hazard
ii. Medical facilities available through employment
iii. Social security, insurance
iv. Sick leave.

Factors in community

i. General description—urban/rural/slum, standard of living
ii. General Attitude of the Community towards disease and patient.

Health care facilities available

i. Availability of voluntary organizations
ii. Leaders in community and their attitudes towards disease
iii. Availability of rehabilitative services
iv. Summary of Salient Social Factors related to the case.

Recommendations

i. Medical management
ii. Changes in Life style for treatment, disability limitation and recurrence of the disease

iii. Physical rehabilitation
iv. Vocational rehabilitation
v. Psychological rehabilitation.

Personality

Personality means certain physical and mental traits which are characteristics of a given individual.

Components

i. Physical. Height, weight, color, etc.
ii. Emotional aspects.
iii. Intelligence.
iv. Behavior, e.g. kind, aggressive, etc.

Determinants

i. Heredity.
ii. **Environment:** Physical (geographical, climatic factors).
iii. **Culture:** The personality of an Indian differs from an Englishman due to differences in culture.
iv. Unique experiences in life.

Personality traits

Cheerful, Manners, sportsmanship, honest, loyal, reliable, sense of humor, kind, tactful, diplomatic, etc.

Types

i. Extrovert
ii. Introvert

Personality disorganization

Individual whose behavior does not conform to the folkways, mores, values and standards of the society is considered a mentally ill with disorganization of his personality.

Causes

a. Excessive stress on the individual (vs. his capabilities)
b. Excessive desires of the individuals
c. Rapid changes in society
d. Heredity factors.

Examples are mentally unwell, alcoholics, drug addicts, prostitutes, destitute, gamblers, criminals, terrorists.

Status and role

Status

In Sociology, status means a position in a group or society. Each status entails some rights to the individual as well as duties. Positions are assigned on the basis of personal characteristics like (age, sex), social activities (leaders), institutional functions (parent, teacher).

i. **Master status:** An individual usually has number of statuses. For example an office clerk is also a husband, father, captain of local football club. When we meet him in his office, his other roles are not visualized by us. The most important status of an individual that basically defines his interaction and relationship with other persons is called Master Status.
ii. **Ascribed status:** Status that one gets by birth or biological characteristics is called ascribed status. Gender, age, caste, family name are examples of ascribed statuses.
iii. **Achieved status:** It is the status that one achieves by his choice, efforts, merit and competition. We become physiotherapists by studying or wife after marriage. Hence these are examples of achieved statuses.

Role

Definition: In sociology, role means expected pattern of behavior. It is the behavior that the society considers appropriate for a given status. For example, the society expects a father to work to earn for maintenance of members of his family. Role is related to status.

Sick role

i. Illness is subjective aspect of disease. It is what the patient feels.
ii. Disease is objective aspect. It is the diagnosis that the doctor makes.
iii. Sickness is the social aspect of ill health.

Sick role is the role expected out of an individual who is not well physically. Following are privileges and duties of a sick person:

i. Exemption from social responsibilities
ii. Privilege of being looked after by others, e.g. family members, society (friends) and Institutions (hospital)
iii. Obligation to seek help for getting better, i.e. treatment, rest, appropriate diet, etc.

Social interaction

Social process: Social process is defined as a social act following another social act, and the following act depending upon the prior act. There are hundreds of social process, important of these are discussed.

Social interaction: Social interactions are key to social life. Without social interactions, there would be no social life, no social group, no society and no culture. Social Interaction can be defined as dynamic interplay of contact between individuals and groups.

Essential requisite of social interaction

a. **Contact:** The contact may be between individuals or groups.

b. **Communication:** Medium is required for communication. Although we can communicate with gestures, but language is the most important means of communication.

Fundamental social processes

a. **Cooperation:** Individuals and groups working together towards a common objective. Example when in class, students discuss a subject among themselves; they have a common aim, i.e. to understand the subject better to do well in examination. Cooperation can be direct or indirect.
b. **Competition:** It is opposite of cooperation. Here individuals or groups compete for common goal. For example, competition among students to get 1st position in class. **Conflict** is also a type of competition and is explained as *competition without rules*. War between countries is an example of conflict.

   We should appreciate that cooperation and competition often coexist. Two students who are the best in class cooperate with each other in discussion on subjects to understand it better, although they are also in competition with each other to win gold medal.
c. **Adjustment:** By adjustment individual or group tries to adjust or fit into what he desires but is not feasible. Parents adjust to demands of their children; students to their teachers.
d. **Accommodation:** Accommodation is a social process of adjustment after conflicts. We see that political parties are in rivalry before elections, but after the results are announced, the leaders of same parties discuss ways to join together to form a government.
e. **Assimilation:** Assimilation is a process by which individuals or groups understands cultural aspects (attitudes, values, etc.) of others individuals or groups. The term is usually

applied to an immigrant or ethnic minority in process of being accepted into a receiving society or ethnically majority.

f. **Isolation:** Isolation is opposite of social contact. It is absence of social contact by individual or group. Isolation is rare, and is considered a negative value.

Medicosocial Problems

chapter

14

Social problems are defined as behavior pattern or conditions that are considered objectionable or undesirable by the society.

Important medicosocial problems are:

i. Juvenile delinquency
ii. Prostitution
iii. Alcohol and drug abuse
iv. Beggary
v. Crimes
vi. Care of handicapped
vii. Care of old people

Juvenile delinquency

Not a new problem, but rapid industrialization and urbanization in recent decades have increased the problem many-folds.

Definition

The Juvenile Justice (Care and Protection of Children) Act, 2000 has defined a "Juvenile in conflict with law" (delinquent) as a juvenile who is alleged to have committed an offence. A 'juvenile' or 'child' means a person who has not completed eighteenth year of age.

Causes

a. **Psychobiological factors:** As per this theory, delinquent children are born delinquent. However, this theory has not many supporters.

b. Environmental factors.
c. Economic factors—Poverty, child labor.
d. Lack of educational facilities.
e. Family Environment e.g. broken or problem families.
f. Bad companionship/neighborhood.
g. Media TV cinema, internet.
h. Exploitation of children by criminals.

Prevention

Proper facilities for children to develop as economically independent human beings. Basic requirement of life, i.e. food, shelter, clothing, education, love and medical care should be met by the community or state, if parents are unable to do so.

Control

i. **Legislative measures:** The Juvenile justice (Care and Protection of Children) Act, 2000 provides a special approach towards care, protection, maintenance, training and rehabilitation of delinquent children. Important provisions under the Act are provision of:
ii. **Probation officers:** Probation officers are appointed to investigate the home/ social conditions of the offenders, observe their conduct, character and health. They submit report to juvenile courts.
iii. **Juvenile courts:** These are special courts for trial of offences committed by children. The purpose is to separate juvenile delinquent from adult criminals.
iv. **Reformatory schools:** These schools are meant for education and vocational training of delinquent children.
v. **Certified and borstal schools:** Children above 16 and below 21 years of age are imparted education and vocational training in Borstal schools.
vi. **Remand homes:** A child under trial is kept in remand home where he is observed for 7–14 days by expert staff

e.g. probation officer, social worker. The experts furnish their report to juvenile courts for decision.

vii. **Foster homes:** For delinquent children under age of 10 years.

ix. **Uncared children institution:** For care of neglected children, orphans, etc.

x. Many of voluntary organizations, religious institutions run many of above institutions. Government provides financial support to these Institutions.

Prostitution

Definition

The practice of habitual intermittent sexual union, more or less promiscuous for mercenary inducement.

Three essential elements of prostitution:

i. Illicit and promiscuous sexual intercourse
ii. Barter, i.e. exchange of money, etc.
iii. Emotional indifference.

Causes

i. **Economic causes:** Poverty and destitution
ii. Illicit sexual relationship
iii. **Domestic causes:** Poverty, broken or problem families
iv. Mental Retardation
v. Desire for easy leisure life
vi. Deception, kidnapping
vii. Devdasi system
viii. Bad influence
ix. In India illiteracy, poverty and ignorance are three basic factors.

Effects

i. **Diseases:** High percentage of sexually-transmitted diseases, e.g. HIV infection, syphilis among prostitutes. Spread of these diseases in community.
ii. **Family disharmony:** Both a cause and result of family disharmony.
iii. Dehumanization of prostitutes.
iv. **Indirect effects:** Crime, alcohol and drug addiction.

Prevention

a. Improving the status of women in society.
b. Education including sex education.
c. More job opportunities for women.
d. Protection and provision of shelter to suppressed/destitute women by Government/Non-Governmental Organization.
e. Legal Measure. Suppression of Immoral Traffic (Prevention) Act, 1956
f. Rehabilitation of prostitutes in community.

Alcoholism and drug dependence

Excessive intake of alcohol leading to medical, social or economic problems is defined as alcoholism.

Drug dependence is psychological or physical need of an individual to periodically intake a drug (chemical) to avoid discomfort that is produced in absence of drug in his/her body system.

Common chemicals being abused

i. Alcohol
ii. Opiates—morphine, heroin
iii. LSD
iv. Cannabis

v. Amphetamines
vi. Tranquilizers or hypnotics (sleep producing drugs), e.g. barbiturates
vii. Cocaine
viii. Tobacco
ix. Volatile solvents
x. Anabolic steroids are also being abused by sportspersons.

Reasons

i. Desire to experiment
ii. Genetic Factors
iii. Seek pleasure especially by depressed or unhappy persons
iv. Social problems, e.g. poverty, chronic stress
v. Broken or problem families
vi. Bad company
vii. Industrialization and urbanization
viii. Unemployment
ix. Living away from homes
x. Migration to cities
xi. Certain occupation, e.g. tourism
xii. Areas with high rates of crimes, prostitution, gambling.

Effects

A. **Effect on Individual**
i. Financial—Loss of money, debt etc.
ii. Loss of status
iii. Loss of job
iv. Health problems—gastritis, liver diseases, impotency, weight gain, neurological problems, heart problems, e.g. hypertension, psychiatric problems
v. Accidents.

B. **Family**
i. Financial hardship

ii. Fights between spouses causing disruption of normal family ties
iii. Broken or problem families
iv. Juvenile delinquency
v. Prostitution
vi. Lack of education of children
vii. Problems in marriages of children
viii. Lack of self respect of family members.

C. **Community**
i. Financial burden on community in form of wastage of human resource
ii. Crimes
iii. Prostitution
iv. Accidents
v. Bad influence on others.

Prevention

a. **Legal approach:** Prohibition of alcohol. Strict legal action against drug peddlers
b. **Educational approach:** Education of students, youth etc.
c. Role of community.
d. Role of social and religious teachers
e. Community should support persons in rehabilitation
f. Organizations like alcohol anonymous.

Treatment

a. Identification of addicts
b. Individual should be motivated to give up drug/alcohol for life
c. Detoxification in hospital settings
d. Post detoxification counseling
e. Follow-up
f. Role of medicosocial worker to identify social cause.

Rehabilitation

Most important and difficult aspect of alcohol and drug dependence. Relapses are very frequent. Comprehensive rehabilitation with medical, social, psychological and vocational rehabilitation should be the aim.

Beggary

i. India has about five lakhs beggars.
ii. Beggars are people who make their living by soliciting alms in public places.

Classification of beggars

i. Child beggars
ii. Physically disabled
iii. Diseased
iv. Able-bodied beggars
v. Religious beggars
vi. Tribal beggars

Causes

a. Unemployment
b. Poverty
c. Disablement or chronic disease
d. Criminal gangs, i.e. criminally organized begging.

Prevention

i. **Legal measures:** Enforcement of law to prevent beggary.
ii. **Social measures:** Support and rehabilitation of beggars.

Crime

Definition

Crime is an act, of commission or omission that is punishable by law of the land.

Causes

i. **Hereditary factors:** Recent studies have refuted this and say that 'crime can not be inherited.'
ii. **Environmental factors:**
   a. Family Environment. Broken or problem families, poverty, alcoholism etc.
   b. Companionship
   c. Education
iii. Economic factors
iv. Role of media especially TV, movies, internet.

Theories of punishment

i. **Retributive theory:** A crime is a wrong committed against humanity, and the offender must pay for it, by undergoing hardship.
ii. **Deterrent theory:** Punishing one criminal, deters others to commit crimes.
iii. **Reformative theory:** This theory aims to see the reasons for carrying out crime by offenders and correct the social pathology behind them. Thus the aim is to prevent crimes, as well reform criminals.

Handicapped child

Now called physically or mentally challenged persons.

Definition

A handicapped child is one who has one or more impairments (anatomical or physiological) that are likely to interfere with normal growth and development or with capacity to learn.

Classification

i. Physically handicapped, e.g. effects of polio, injury, burns etc.

ii. Visually handicapped
iii. Hearing impairment
iv. Speech defects
v. Cerebral palsy
vi. Mental Retardation
vii. Socially handicapped. Extreme poverty, low caste, orphans.

Causes

i. **Genetic conditions:** Down's Syndrome
ii. **Antenatal causes:** Rubella infection during pregnancy
iii. **Perinatal causes:** Injury during child birth
iv. **Post natal causes:** Infection, accidents
v. **Other causes:** Malnutrition, late pregnancy

Prevention

Primary prevention

i. Genetic counseling
ii. Immunization, e.g. Rubella vaccination, oral polio vaccine
iii. Nutrition, e.g. prevention of deficiency of iodine
iv. Care of mothers and children through maternal and child health services.

Secondary prevention

i. Early diagnosis of impairment
ii. Proper treatment
iii. **Training and education:** Speech therapy, training for blind, special schools, etc.

Rehabilitation

i. **Vocational training:** Work and improve with what is left
ii. Reservation of jobs for handicapped.

Health problem of the aged

Due to better nutrition, environment and health care, we are living longer, increasing the percentage of old people in developed and developing countries. In India about 7.2 percent of people are above the age of 60 years.

Problems

Physical

All the organs and systems do not function properly.

i. **Eye:** Low vision due to cataract, glaucoma
ii. Hearing loss
iii. Dental and gum diseases
iv. **Heart problems:** hypertension, coronary artery disease (CAD)
v. **CNS:** Loss of memory, cerebral stroke
vi. Cancers
vii. Accidents
viii. **Joint problems:** Osteoarthritis, rheumatoid arthritis, gait defects
ix. **Respiratory diseases:** COPD, Asthma
x. **Genitourinary problems:** Prostrate, incontinence of urine
xi. **Gynecological problems:** Prolapse of uterus.

Psychological

Lack of company especially if spouse has died or separated, generation gap, loneliness, depression.

Economic

i. Poverty
ii. Increase expenditure on drugs, etc.

Health aging: what can be done?

i. **Nutrition:** Healthy and balanced diet.
ii. Exercise
iii. Weight control
iv. Smoking to be stopped
v. Alcohol intake within limits
vi. **Social activities:** Old age groups
vii. Diagnosis of diseases and early treatment to prevent complications
viii. **Social support:** Involvement of aged in social activities; and involvement of young in care of elderly.

Index